Hiatal Hernia Diet Guide for Beginners

The Importance of Diet for Hiatal Hernia

By

Jamie Louden

Table of Contents

CHAPTER 1

Introduction

1.1 What is a Hiatal Hernia?

A hiatal hernia, also known as a hiatus hernia, is a medical condition that occurs when a portion of the stomach protrudes through the diaphragm and into the chest cavity. To fully grasp the nature of this condition, it's essential to understand the anatomy involved. The diaphragm is a muscular wall that separates the chest cavity from the abdominal cavity. Its primary role is to assist in the process of breathing. Just above the diaphragm is an opening called the esophageal hiatus, through which the esophagus passes before connecting to the stomach.

In the case of a hiatal hernia, a part of the stomach, usually the upper portion, pushes through this opening and enters the chest cavity. This displacement can lead to a range of symptoms, primarily related to gastroesophageal reflux, which is the backflow of stomach acid and other gastric contents into the esophagus. This reflux can cause irritation and inflammation of the esophagus, resulting in symptoms like heartburn, regurgitation, chest pain, and difficulty swallowing.

Hiatal hernias can be categorized into two main types:

1. **Sliding Hiatal Hernia:** This is the most common type of hiatal hernia. In a sliding hiatal

hernia, the junction where the esophagus meets the stomach and part of the stomach itself move up into the chest. The position of the junction and the extent of herniation can vary.

2. **Paraesophageal Hiatal Hernia:** This type is less common but can be more serious. In a paraesophageal hiatal hernia, a portion of the stomach pushes through the diaphragm alongside the esophagus. Unlike a sliding hernia, the esophagus remains in its normal position, and this type is more likely to cause complications like gastric strangulation or obstruction.

Hiatal hernias can be caused by a combination of factors, including age, obesity, smoking, and genetics. They can develop gradually over time or occur suddenly due to factors such as heavy lifting, sudden physical exertion, or trauma. While hiatal hernias can affect people of all ages, they are more common in individuals over the age of 50.

1.2 The Importance of Diet for Hiatal Hernia

Understanding the importance of diet in the context of hiatal hernia is crucial for managing this condition effectively. Diet plays a significant role in alleviating symptoms, preventing complications, and improving the overall quality of life for individuals with hiatal hernias. Here are several key reasons why diet is of paramount importance:

A. Symptom Management: Diet can help in the management of common symptoms associated with hiatal hernia, particularly gastroesophageal reflux disease (GERD). GERD is characterized by symptoms like heartburn, regurgitation, chest pain, and difficulty swallowing. By making appropriate dietary choices, individuals can reduce the frequency and severity of these symptoms.

B. Minimizing Acid Reflux: Certain foods and dietary habits can trigger or exacerbate acid reflux, which is a hallmark of hiatal hernia. By avoiding these triggers and making informed choices about what they eat and when they eat, individuals can reduce the occurrence of acid reflux episodes.

C. Weight Management: Obesity is a known risk factor for the development and worsening of hiatal hernias. Maintaining a healthy weight through diet and exercise can reduce the pressure on the abdominal area, which, in turn, can help prevent the stomach from pushing through the diaphragm.

D. Preventing Complications: Hiatal hernias can lead to complications such as esophagitis (inflammation of the esophagus), Barrett's esophagus (a precancerous condition), and even esophageal cancer. A proper diet can contribute to reducing the risk of these complications by minimizing the exposure of the esophagus to stomach acid.

E. Enhancing Overall Health: A diet designed for hiatal hernia management can also have broader health benefits. It can promote good digestion, maintain a healthy gastrointestinal tract, and support overall well-being. Choosing the right foods can improve nutritional intake, energy levels, and the body's ability to heal and recover.

In essence, the significance of diet in the context of hiatal hernia is multi-faceted. It encompasses symptom relief, prevention of complications, and the promotion of general health. By following a well-informed hiatal hernia diet plan, individuals can take an active role in managing their condition and enjoying an improved quality of life. It's important to remember that dietary recommendations may vary from person to person, so consulting with a healthcare professional or a registered dietitian is often recommended to tailor a diet plan to individual needs and preferences.

CHAPTER 2

Understanding Hiatal Hernia

2.1 What Causes a Hiatal Hernia?

Understanding the underlying causes of hiatal hernias is essential to appreciate how this condition develops. Hiatal hernias can be caused by a combination of factors, and while the exact cause can vary from person to person, there are several common contributors:

1. **Age:** Age is a significant factor in the development of hiatal hernias. As people age, the muscles and tissues that support

the diaphragm may weaken, making it easier for the stomach to herniate through the diaphragmatic opening.

2. **Obesity:** Excess weight, especially around the abdominal area, can increase the pressure on the stomach and the diaphragm. This added pressure can lead to a higher likelihood of a hiatal hernia developing or worsening.

3. **Genetics:** There may be a genetic predisposition to hiatal hernias. If close family members, such as parents or siblings, have had hiatal hernias, an individual may have an increased risk.

4. **Pregnancy:** Pregnant women can experience increased intra-

abdominal pressure due to the growing uterus. This pressure can contribute to the development of a hiatal hernia or exacerbate an existing one.

5. **Heavy Lifting or Straining:** Activities that involve heavy lifting or straining, such as weightlifting or constipation, can raise intra-abdominal pressure, potentially causing a hiatal hernia, particularly in those with weakened diaphragmatic support.

6. **Smoking:** Smoking is associated with a higher risk of developing hiatal hernias. It can weaken the lower esophageal sphincter (LES), the muscular ring that separates the esophagus from the stomach, which plays a crucial role in

preventing stomach acid from flowing back into the esophagus.

7. **Trauma or Injury:** Trauma to the chest or abdomen, such as from a car accident or a severe blow to the upper abdomen, can result in a hiatal hernia.

It's important to note that hiatal hernias can develop gradually over time or occur suddenly due to various factors. While these factors increase the risk, not everyone exposed to them will develop a hiatal hernia. Additionally, the risk factors and causes can vary depending on the type of hiatal hernia.

2.2 Types of Hiatal Hernias

Hiatal hernias can be categorized into two primary types:

1. **Sliding Hiatal Hernia:** This is the most common type of hiatal hernia. In a sliding hiatal hernia, the gastroesophageal junction (where the esophagus connects to the stomach) and a portion of the stomach itself move up into the chest through the esophageal hiatus in the diaphragm. The extent of herniation can vary, with some cases involving only a slight displacement, while others may involve a more significant portion of the stomach moving into the chest.

2. **Paraesophageal Hiatal Hernia:** This type is less common but can be more serious. In a paraesophageal hiatal hernia, a portion of the stomach moves through the diaphragm next to the esophagus, while the gastroesophageal junction remains in its normal position. This type of hernia is more likely to cause complications, as it can result in gastric strangulation, which is when blood flow to the herniated portion of the stomach is compromised.

2.3 Symptoms and Complications

The symptoms of a hiatal hernia can vary depending on the type and severity of the hernia. Common symptoms associated with hiatal hernias include:

- **Heartburn:** A burning sensation in the chest, often accompanied by sour or acidic taste in the mouth.

- **Regurgitation:** The backflow of stomach contents into the esophagus, sometimes leading to the sensation of food or liquid coming back up.

- **Chest Pain:** Some individuals experience chest pain or discomfort, which can be mistaken for heart-related issues.

- **Difficulty Swallowing:** Hiatal hernias can lead to difficulty in swallowing, known as dysphagia, especially when the hernia compresses the esophagus.

- **Belching:** Excessive belching or burping can occur due to increased pressure on the stomach.

- **Nausea:** Nausea and an upset stomach can be common symptoms.

Complications associated with hiatal hernias can include:

- **Esophagitis:** Inflammation of the esophagus caused by the backflow of stomach acid, which can lead to pain and discomfort.

- **Barrett's Esophagus:** A condition in which the lining of the esophagus changes due to repeated exposure to stomach acid, increasing the risk of esophageal cancer.

- **Gastric Strangulation:** In paraesophageal hiatal hernias, the stomach can become twisted or pinched, leading to reduced blood flow and potentially requiring emergency surgery.

It's important to note that not everyone with a hiatal hernia experiences symptoms, and some individuals may have hiatal hernias discovered incidentally during medical tests for other conditions.

Treatment and management of hiatal hernias typically focus on relieving symptoms, preventing complications, and improving overall quality of life.

CHAPTER 3

Dietary Guidelines for Hiatal Hernia

3.1 General Diet Recommendations

Maintaining a well-balanced diet is crucial for managing the symptoms and complications associated with a hiatal hernia. Here are some general dietary recommendations to consider:

1. **Small, Frequent Meals:** Instead of three large meals a day, opt for smaller, more frequent meals. This can help reduce the pressure on the

stomach and minimize the risk of acid reflux.

2. **Chew Thoroughly:** Take your time to chew your food thoroughly. This aids digestion and reduces the risk of overeating.

3. **Eat Slowly:** Eating slowly and mindfully can prevent swallowing air, which can lead to bloating and gas.

4. **Stay Upright After Eating:** Avoid lying down immediately after a meal. Instead, remain upright or engage in light physical activity to aid digestion and minimize the risk of reflux.

5. **Stay Hydrated:** Drink plenty of water throughout the day, but avoid excessive fluid intake

during meals, as this can increase stomach pressure.

6. **Incorporate Fiber:** Include high-fiber foods like whole grains, fruits, and vegetables in your diet to promote regular bowel movements and prevent constipation.

7. **Lean Proteins:** Opt for lean sources of protein, such as poultry, fish, tofu, and legumes, while limiting fatty or fried meats.

8. **Low-Fat Dairy:** Choose low-fat or fat-free dairy products to reduce the risk of triggering reflux.

9. **Complex Carbohydrates:** Consume complex carbohydrates like whole grains, rice, and pasta, which

are less likely to cause reflux compared to high-fat or spicy foods.

10. **Non-Citrus Fruits:** Enjoy non-citrus fruits like apples, pears, and bananas, which are less acidic and less likely to trigger reflux.

11. **Vegetables:** Most vegetables are well-tolerated, but be mindful of gas-producing options like broccoli, cauliflower, and cabbage.

12. **Ginger and Chamomile Tea:** These herbal teas are known for their soothing properties and can be helpful for digestion.

3.2 Foods to Avoid

To reduce the risk of acid reflux and other symptoms associated with hiatal hernias, it's important to avoid or limit the consumption of the following foods and beverages:

1. **Citrus Fruits:** Oranges, grapefruits, lemons, and other citrus fruits are highly acidic and can trigger reflux.

2. **Tomatoes and Tomato Products:** Tomato-based foods like pasta sauce, ketchup, and salsa can be problematic due to their acidity.

3. **Spicy Foods:** Spices, hot peppers, and spicy dishes can exacerbate heartburn and reflux.

4. **Fatty and Fried Foods:** High-fat foods, such as fried foods, fatty cuts of meat, and full-fat dairy products, can relax the lower esophageal sphincter (LES), leading to increased reflux.

5. **Mint and Peppermint:** These can relax the LES and may contribute to acid reflux symptoms.

6. **Chocolate:** Chocolate contains substances that can relax the LES and may trigger reflux.

7. **Caffeine:** Coffee, tea, and caffeinated beverages can increase stomach acid production and contribute to reflux.

8. **Alcohol:** Alcoholic beverages can relax the LES and irritate

the esophagus, making reflux
more likely.

9. **Carbonated Beverages:**
    Carbonated drinks, including
    soda, can lead to gas and
    bloating, which can worsen
    symptoms.

10. **Onions and Garlic:** These
    foods can relax the LES and
    may contribute to heartburn.

11. **Peppermint:** Peppermint can
    relax the LES, potentially
    leading to reflux.

12. **Processed Foods:** Highly
    processed and pre-packaged
    foods often contain additives
    and preservatives that can
    trigger reflux.

13. **Acidic and Carbonated
    Drinks:** Avoid drinks like

citrus juices, carbonated sodas, and sports drinks that can be irritating to the esophagus.

Individual responses to specific foods can vary, so it's essential to pay attention to your body and identify personal triggers. Additionally, it's advisable to consult with a healthcare professional or a registered dietitian to create a personalized diet plan that addresses your specific dietary needs and helps manage your hiatal hernia effectively.

3.3 Foods to Include

Incorporating the right foods into your diet can help manage hiatal hernia symptoms and promote better digestive health. Here are some foods to include in your hiatal hernia-friendly diet:

1. **Lean Proteins:** Choose lean sources of protein like skinless poultry, fish, tofu, legumes, and lean cuts of beef or pork. These options are less likely to trigger reflux.

2. **Complex Carbohydrates:** Opt for whole grains like brown rice, whole wheat pasta, quinoa, and oatmeal. These foods are generally better tolerated than high-fat or spicy options.

3. **Non-Citrus Fruits:** Enjoy fruits like apples, pears, bananas, and melons, which are less acidic and less likely to cause reflux.

4. **Vegetables:** Most vegetables are well-tolerated and can be included in your diet. Focus on

green, leafy vegetables and non-gassy options.

5. **Ginger:** Fresh ginger can have soothing properties and is known to aid digestion. Incorporate it into your meals or brew ginger tea.

6. **Chamomile Tea:** Chamomile tea is often used for its calming and digestive benefits. It can be a helpful beverage choice.

7. **Low-Fat Dairy:** opt for low-fat or fat-free dairy products like milk, yogurt, and cheese. These are less likely to trigger reflux compared to full-fat options.

8. **Herbs:** Use herbs like basil, oregano, and parsley to add flavor to your meals without adding excessive spice.

9. **Egg Whites:** Egg whites are a good source of protein and can be included in your diet.

10. **Oatmeal:** Oatmeal is a soothing and easily digestible breakfast option. You can add non-citrus fruits and a touch of honey for flavor.

11. **Banana Smoothies:** Blend a banana with non-citrus fruits and low-fat yogurt to create a nutritious and reflux-friendly smoothie.

12. **Poultry or Tofu Stir-Fries:** Create stir-fries with lean protein sources and plenty of vegetables for a balanced meal.

3.4 Portion Control and Meal Frequency

In addition to selecting the right foods, paying attention to portion control and meal frequency can be highly beneficial for individuals with hiatal hernias:

1. **Portion Control:** Be mindful of portion sizes. Eating large meals can put added pressure on the stomach and increase the risk of reflux. Consider using smaller plates and bowls to help control portion sizes.

2. **Meal Frequency:** Instead of consuming three large meals a day, aim for smaller, more frequent meals. This approach can help prevent overeating and reduce the risk of symptoms

like heartburn and
regurgitation.

3. **Snacking:** Healthy, balanced snacks can help maintain energy levels and prevent excessive hunger. Opt for nutrient-dense snacks like a handful of almonds, a piece of fruit, or yogurt.

4. **Avoid Late-Night Eating:** Try to finish eating at least two to three hours before bedtime to minimize the risk of nighttime reflux.

5. **Stay Upright After Eating:** After meals, remain in an upright position to allow food to digest properly. Lying down immediately after eating can increase the likelihood of reflux.

6. **Hydration:** Stay well-hydrated throughout the day, but be cautious about excessive fluid intake during meals, as it can increase stomach pressure.

7. **Chewing and Savoring:** Chew your food thoroughly and savor each bite. Eating slowly and mindfully can help prevent overeating and promote good digestion.

Individual dietary preferences and tolerances can vary, so it's important to find a routine and meal plan that works best for you. Consulting with a healthcare professional or a registered dietitian can provide personalized guidance to help manage your hiatal hernia effectively through diet.

CHAPTER 4

Sample Hiatal Hernia Diet Plan

4.1 Breakfast Ideas

Start your day with a nutritious and reflux-friendly breakfast. Here are some breakfast ideas for individuals with hiatal hernias:

Option 1: Oatmeal Delight

- 1/2 cup of old-fashioned oats

- Sliced bananas or berries (non-citrus)

- 1-2 tablespoons of honey or maple syrup for sweetness

- A sprinkle of ground flaxseeds for added fiber

- A cup of chamomile tea or ginger tea

Option 2: Greek Yogurt Parfait

- 6 oz of low-fat Greek yogurt

- Sliced non-citrus fruits like strawberries or kiwi

- A handful of granola (choose a low-fat, low-sugar option)

- A drizzle of honey for added sweetness

- Herbal tea or a glass of water

Option 3: Scrambled Eggs and Toast

- Scrambled eggs made with egg whites (2-3 egg whites)

- Whole-grain toast or a whole-grain English muffin

- Sautéed spinach or other non-citrus vegetables

- Herbal tea or water

Option 4: Peanut Butter and Banana Toast

- Whole-grain toast

- A thin spread of natural peanut butter

- Sliced banana

- A touch of honey for extra flavor

- Herbal tea or water

4.2 Lunch Suggestions

Lunch is an opportunity to maintain a balanced diet while keeping hiatal hernia symptoms in check. Here are some lunch ideas:

Option 1: Grilled Chicken Salad

- Grilled, skinless chicken breast

- Mixed greens or spinach

- Sliced non-citrus vegetables like cucumber, bell peppers, and carrots

- Balsamic vinaigrette dressing (in moderation)

- A whole-grain roll or breadstick

- Water or herbal tea

Option 2: Tuna Salad Wrap

- Tuna salad made with light mayonnaise or Greek yogurt

- Whole-grain tortilla or wrap

- Lettuce, tomato, and non-citrus veggies

- Sliced avocado for creaminess

- A side of non-citrus fruit salad

- Water or herbal tea

Option 3: Quinoa and Vegetable Bowl

- Cooked quinoa

- Sautéed or roasted non-citrus vegetables like zucchini, broccoli, and sweet potatoes

- A source of lean protein, such as tofu or beans

- A drizzle of olive oil and herbs for flavor

- A small serving of yogurt with honey for dessert

- Water or herbal tea

Option 4: Baked Sweet Potato with Cottage Cheese

- Baked sweet potato topped with low-fat cottage cheese

- Steamed or sautéed non-citrus vegetables

- A side of mixed berries (non-citrus)

- Herbal tea or water

These breakfast and lunch ideas provide a good starting point for your hiatal hernia diet plan. Remember to adjust portion sizes to your specific needs, and feel free to customize your meals based on your taste preferences and dietary requirements. Additionally, stay hydrated throughout the day and aim for small, frequent meals to help manage your hiatal hernia effectively.

4.3 Dinner Options

Dinner can be a satisfying and reflux-friendly meal with the right choices. Here are some dinner options for individuals with hiatal hernias:

Option 1: Baked Salmon with Brown Rice

- Baked or grilled salmon (rich in omega-3 fatty acids)

- Brown rice or quinoa

- Steamed or roasted non-citrus vegetables like broccoli and asparagus

- A light olive oil drizzle with herbs for flavor

- Water or herbal tea

Option 2: Veggie Stir-Fry

- Stir-fried tofu or skinless chicken breast

- A variety of non-citrus vegetables like bell peppers, snow peas, and bok choy

- A low-sodium, reflux-friendly stir-fry sauce

- Served over brown rice or whole-grain noodles

- A side of sliced melon (non-citrus)

- Water or herbal tea

Option 3: Turkey and Avocado Wrap

- Lean ground turkey or turkey breast slices

- Whole-grain tortilla or wrap

- Sliced avocado, lettuce, and tomato

- A light, non-citrus vinaigrette for dressing

- Steamed or roasted non-citrus vegetables as a side

- Water or herbal tea

Option 4: Quinoa Stuffed Peppers

- Bell peppers filled with a quinoa and vegetable mixture

- A source of lean protein like ground turkey or black beans

- Baked until the peppers are tender

- A small serving of non-citrus fruit salad for dessert

- Water or herbal tea

4.4 Snacks for Hiatal Hernia

Healthy snacks can keep your energy levels up and prevent excessive hunger between meals. Here are some hiatal hernia-friendly snack ideas:

Option 1: Greek Yogurt and Berries

- A small serving of low-fat Greek yogurt

- Fresh, non-citrus berries like strawberries or blueberries

- A drizzle of honey for sweetness (optional)

Option 2: Rice Cakes with Hummus

- Whole-grain rice cakes

- Hummus for dipping

- Sliced cucumber or carrot sticks

Option 3: Cottage Cheese and Pineapple

- Low-fat cottage cheese

- Chunks of fresh pineapple (ensure it's ripe and non-acidic)

- A sprinkle of cinnamon for flavor

Option 4: Almonds and Dried Apricots

- A small handful of raw almonds

- Dried apricots (ensure they are unsulfured and unsweetened)

Option 5: Smoothie

- A homemade smoothie made with non-citrus fruits, like bananas and berries

- Low-fat yogurt or almond milk

- A touch of honey for sweetness (optional)

Portion control is key, even with snacks. It's also important to listen to your body and avoid overeating. If you experience any discomfort or symptoms, adjust your dietary choices accordingly. Staying hydrated with water or reflux-friendly herbal teas between meals can also be helpful for maintaining overall digestive health.

CHAPTER 5

Beverages and Hiatal Hernia

5.1 Hydration and Hiatal Hernia

Hydration is essential for overall health, and it's particularly important for individuals with hiatal hernias. Proper hydration can help with digestion, prevent constipation, and support overall well-being. Here are some guidelines for staying hydrated with a hiatal hernia:

- **Drink Small Sips:** Instead of gulping large amounts of fluids at once, sip water or other beverages slowly in small quantities to avoid increasing stomach pressure.

- **Avoid Excessive Fluids During Meals:** While it's important to stay hydrated, avoid excessive fluid intake during meals, as this can dilute stomach acid and potentially lead to reflux. It's better to consume most of your fluids between meals.

- **Stay Hydrated Throughout the Day:** Drink water or reflux-friendly beverages between meals to ensure proper hydration. Herbal teas, water, and non-acidic juices are good options.

- **Herbal Teas:** Consider herbal teas like chamomile or ginger tea. These can have soothing properties and may help with digestion.

- **Limit Caffeinated and Carbonated Beverages:** Caffeine can increase stomach acid production, potentially leading to reflux. Carbonated beverages, including soda, can cause gas and bloating. If you consume these, do so in moderation.

- **Alcohol:** Alcohol can relax the lower esophageal sphincter (LES), which can lead to increased reflux. If you choose to consume alcohol, do so in moderation.

5.2 Safe and Problematic Beverages

Here's a breakdown of safe and problematic beverages for individuals with hiatal hernias:

Safe Beverages:

1. **Water:** Plain water is the best choice for staying hydrated. It does not increase stomach pressure or contribute to reflux.

2. **Herbal Teas:** Herbal teas like chamomile, ginger, and peppermint can have soothing properties that may help with digestion and minimize reflux symptoms.

3. **Non-Citrus Juices:** Non-citrus juices like apple, pear, or melon juice are generally well-

tolerated and less likely to trigger reflux.

4. **Non-Carbonated Water with a Twist:** Adding a twist of lemon or lime to non-carbonated water can be a safe way to infuse flavor without triggering reflux for some individuals.

Problematic Beverages:

1. **Citrus Juices:** Citrus juices like orange, grapefruit, and lemon are highly acidic and can trigger reflux symptoms.

2. **Caffeinated Beverages:** Coffee, regular tea, and caffeinated sodas can increase stomach acid production and contribute to reflux.

3. **Carbonated Beverages:**
    Carbonated sodas, sparkling
    water, and other fizzy drinks
    can cause gas and bloating,
    which may exacerbate hiatal
    hernia symptoms.

4. **Alcohol:** Alcohol, especially in
    excess, can relax the LES,
    potentially leading to increased
    reflux symptoms.

5. **Mint Tea:** While peppermint
    tea is generally considered safe
    for some individuals, it can
    relax the LES in others and
    worsen symptoms.

It's important to remember that
individual responses to beverages can
vary, so it's crucial to pay attention to
your body and identify personal
triggers. If you experience discomfort
or increased reflux after consuming

specific beverages, it's advisable to limit or avoid them. Consult with a healthcare professional or a registered dietitian to create a personalized dietary plan that best suits your needs and helps manage your hiatal hernia effectively.

CHAPTER 6

Eating Habits for Hiatal Hernia Relief

6.1 Slow and Mindful Eating

Eating habits play a significant role in managing hiatal hernia symptoms, and adopting a slow and mindful approach to eating can be particularly beneficial. Here's why and how to incorporate this practice into your daily routine:

Why Slow and Mindful Eating Helps:

- **Prevents Overeating:** Eating slowly allows your body to register fullness, reducing the risk of overeating, which can put added pressure on the stomach and trigger reflux.

- **Better Digestion:** Chewing your food thoroughly initiates the digestive process in the mouth and makes it easier for your stomach to break down the food.

- **Minimizes Air Swallowing:** Rushed eating often leads to swallowing excess air, which can cause bloating and gas. Eating slowly helps prevent this.

- **Enjoyment of Food:** Mindful eating allows you to savor and enjoy your meals, which can enhance your overall dining experience.

How to Eat Slowly and Mindfully:

1. **Chew Thoroughly:** Take your time to chew each bite thoroughly. Aim for at least 20-30 chews per bite. This practice aids digestion and prevents overeating.

2. **Put Down Utensils:** Set down your utensils between bites. This simple act encourages you to pause and savor your food.

3. **Engage Your Senses:** Pay attention to the flavors, textures, and aromas of your food. Fully engage your senses in the eating experience.

4. **Small Bites:** Take smaller, manageable bites to help control portion sizes and promote mindful eating.

5. **No Distractions:** Eat without distractions, such as watching

TV, working on the computer, or scrolling through your phone. Focus on your meal.

6. **Take Breaks:** Pause during your meal to check in with your hunger levels. Are you still hungry, or are you satisfied? This practice can help prevent overeating.

6.2 Proper Posture

Proper posture while eating can also contribute to hiatal hernia relief and improved digestion. Here's how the right posture can make a difference:

Why Proper Posture Matters:

- **Minimizes Pressure:** Maintaining an upright posture while eating helps prevent increased intra-abdominal pressure. This, in turn, reduces the risk of stomach contents moving into the chest cavity.

- **Supports Digestion:** Good posture aligns your digestive organs, allowing them to function optimally and ensuring proper movement of food through your digestive system.

- **Reduces Discomfort:** Proper posture can minimize discomfort and the likelihood of experiencing symptoms like heartburn, regurgitation, and bloating.

How to Maintain Proper Posture While Eating:

1. **Sit Upright:** Whether you're at a table or eating on the couch, sit up straight with your back

against the chair and feet flat on the floor.

2. **Use Support:** If possible, use a dining chair with proper back support to encourage good posture.

3. **Avoid Slouching:** Refrain from slouching or hunching over your food. Keep your spine straight.

4. **Elbows on the Table:** Rest your elbows on the table to support your upper body, but keep your back straight.

5. **Take Your Time:** Eating slowly and mindfully goes hand in hand with proper posture. Avoid leaning over your plate while rushing through your meal.

6. **Sit for a While After Eating:**
Remain in an upright position
for at least 30 minutes after
eating to allow food to digest
properly and reduce the risk of
reflux.

By practicing slow and mindful eating
with proper posture, you can make
significant strides in managing hiatal
hernia symptoms and improving your
overall eating experience. These
habits are simple yet effective ways to
promote digestive health and
minimize discomfort associated with
hiatal hernias.

6.3 Avoiding Overeating

Avoiding overeating is essential for
individuals with hiatal hernias.
Overeating can increase the pressure
on the stomach and lead to more

frequent and severe reflux symptoms. Here are some strategies to help you avoid overeating:

- **Portion Control:** Use smaller plates and bowls to control portion sizes. When dining out, consider sharing a meal or taking leftovers home.

- **Chew Thoroughly:** As mentioned earlier, chewing your food thoroughly can help you slow down and recognize when you're full, reducing the risk of overeating.

- **Listen to Your Body:** Pay attention to your body's hunger and fullness cues. Eat until you're comfortably satisfied, not overly full.

- **Eat Mindfully:** Avoid eating in front of the TV or while distracted. Focus on your meal, savor the flavors, and engage your senses.

- **Use a Timer:** If you tend to eat too quickly, set a timer for 20-30 minutes for each meal. Try to extend your mealtime to allow for proper digestion and prevent overeating.

- **Avoid Emotional Eating:** Try to differentiate between physical hunger and emotional hunger. Don't use food as a way to cope with stress, boredom, or other emotions.

6.4 Timing of Meals

The timing of your meals can impact hiatal hernia symptoms, especially the timing of your last meal before bedtime. Here are some guidelines for meal timing:

- **Finish Early:** Try to finish your last meal at least two to three hours before going to bed. This allows time for digestion and reduces the likelihood of nighttime reflux.

- **Evening Snacks:** If you find that you need a snack before bedtime, choose a light and reflux-friendly option. Consider a small serving of non-citrus fruit, a small handful of almonds, or a slice of whole-grain bread with a bit of peanut butter.

- **Consistent Meal Timing:** Try to establish a regular schedule for meals. Consistency in meal timing can help regulate your digestion and reduce the risk of overeating.

- **Balanced Breakfast:** Don't skip breakfast, and aim to have a substantial, balanced meal in the morning. This can help prevent excessive hunger later in the day, which might lead to overeating.

- **Moderate Evening Meals:** While it's advisable to have a lighter meal in the evening, ensure that it's still nutritionally balanced. Avoid large, heavy dinners that may lead to discomfort or reflux.

- **Stay Upright:** After your last meal, remain in an upright position to allow time for digestion before lying down or going to bed.

paying attention to the timing of your meals and practicing portion control, you can significantly reduce the risk of overeating and improve the management of hiatal hernia symptoms, particularly nighttime reflux. Listening to your body's cues and maintaining a consistent meal schedule can promote better digestive health and overall well-being.

CHAPTER 7

Cooking Tips for Hiatal Hernia-Friendly Meals

7.1 Cooking Methods

Choosing the right cooking methods can make a significant difference when preparing hiatal hernia-friendly meals. Here are some cooking methods to consider:

Baking: Baking is a gentle cooking method that doesn't require the addition of excessive fats or oils. It's suitable for preparing lean proteins like chicken, turkey, fish, and tofu, as well as vegetables. You can bake dishes like chicken breasts with herbs and vegetables for a flavorful and reflux-friendly meal.

Grilling: Grilling is a healthy way to prepare food, especially when you use lean cuts of meat, poultry, or fish. Season with reflux-friendly herbs and spices, and avoid high-fat marinades. Grilled vegetables can also be a delicious and well-tolerated side dish.

Steaming: Steaming is an excellent method for preserving the nutritional value of vegetables. Steamed broccoli, carrots, or cauliflower can make a nutritious addition to your meals.

Sautéing: When sautéing, use a small amount of heart-healthy olive oil or canola oil. Sauté lean proteins and non-citrus vegetables with mild seasonings to keep the dish reflux-friendly.

Poaching: Poaching is a gentle cooking method where you simmer food in liquid. It's suitable for cooking chicken or fish. Poached chicken can be used in various dishes, from salads to wraps.

Slow Cooking: Slow cookers or crockpots can be a convenient way to prepare reflux-friendly meals. Use lean proteins, non-citrus vegetables, and mild seasonings to create flavorful and easily digestible dishes.

Blending and Pureeing: For individuals with difficulty swallowing due to hiatal hernia symptoms, blending or pureeing foods can be helpful. This can turn whole meals into smoother, more easily consumed textures.

Boiling: Boiling is a simple method for cooking pasta, rice, and certain vegetables. Choose whole grains and non-citrus vegetables to keep your meal reflux-friendly.

7.2 Seasonings and Flavorings

Seasonings and flavorings can add zest to your hiatal hernia-friendly meals without causing discomfort. Here are some options to consider:

- **Herbs:** Use fresh or dried herbs like basil, oregano, parsley, thyme, and rosemary to season your dishes. Herbs add flavor without the need for excessive salt or spice.

- **Spices:** Some mild spices like cinnamon, nutmeg, and cardamom can be well-tolerated and add a hint of warmth and flavor to your meals. Avoid very spicy spices like cayenne or chili powder.

- **Garlic and Ginger:** Fresh or powdered garlic and ginger can be used to enhance the flavor of your dishes without causing reflux symptoms. These ingredients can be soothing to the stomach.

- **Lemon or Lime Zest:** While citrus juice can be problematic for reflux, using small amounts of lemon or lime zest to season your food can add a burst of flavor without the acidity.

- **Olive Oil:** Use heart-healthy olive oil or canola oil for sautéing and as a mild salad dressing. It adds richness to your dishes without triggering reflux.

- **Balsamic Vinegar:** A drizzle of balsamic vinegar, used in moderation, can add depth and flavor to salads and dishes.

- **Low-Sodium Broths:** Use low-sodium chicken or vegetable broths to add flavor and moisture to your cooking without excess salt.

- **Low-Fat Yogurt:** Low-fat yogurt can be used as a base for sauces, marinades, or salad dressings. It adds creaminess without excess fat.

Experiment with these cooking methods and seasonings to create a variety of delicious and reflux-friendly meals. Tailor your recipes to your preferences and dietary needs, and pay attention to how your body responds to different ingredients to make the best choices for managing hiatal hernia symptoms.

CHAPTER 8

Managing Hiatal Hernia Symptoms

8.1 Heartburn and Acid Reflux

Heartburn and acid reflux are common symptoms of hiatal hernias. To manage these symptoms effectively, consider the following strategies:

- **Dietary Modifications:** As discussed in previous sections, adhere to a hiatal hernia-friendly diet. Avoid trigger foods, such as citrus fruits, spicy dishes, and fatty foods. Focus on smaller, more frequent meals to reduce the pressure on the stomach and minimize reflux.

- **Elevate Your Upper Body:** Elevating the head of your bed by about 6-8 inches can help prevent stomach acid from flowing into the esophagus while you sleep. Alternatively, use extra pillows to prop yourself up.

- **Avoid Lying Down After Meals:** After eating, remain in an upright position for at least 2-3 hours to allow food to digest properly and reduce the risk of reflux.

- **Wear Loose Clothing:** Tight clothing around your waist can increase pressure on your stomach, potentially worsening heartburn and reflux symptoms. Opt for loose-fitting attire.

- **Antacids:** Over-the-counter antacids can provide temporary relief from heartburn. However, consult with a healthcare professional before using them regularly.

- **Medications:** If lifestyle changes and dietary adjustments are insufficient, your healthcare provider may prescribe medications such as proton pump inhibitors (PPIs) or H2 receptor blockers to reduce stomach acid production. Follow your healthcare provider's recommendations regarding medication usage.

8.2 Regurgitation

Regurgitation is the sensation of food or stomach contents moving back into the throat or mouth. To manage this symptom:

- **Stay Upright:** After meals, stay in an upright position for at least 2-3 hours to promote proper digestion and minimize the risk of regurgitation.

- **Avoid Overeating:** Overeating can increase the risk of regurgitation. Practice portion control and eat slowly to prevent overconsumption.

- **Mindful Chewing:** Chew your food thoroughly, as this can help reduce the risk of regurgitation. Eating mindfully can also aid digestion.

- **Elevate Your Upper Body:** As mentioned earlier, elevate the head of your bed or use extra pillows to sleep at an incline. This position can help prevent stomach contents from flowing back into the throat.

- **Medications:** In some cases, medications to reduce stomach acid production may help alleviate regurgitation symptoms. Consult with a healthcare professional for guidance.

8.3 Bloating and Gas

Bloating and gas can be uncomfortable side effects of hiatal hernias. To manage these symptoms:

- **Dietary Adjustments:** Avoid gas-producing foods like beans, lentils, broccoli, cauliflower, and cabbage. Also, limit carbonated beverages, which can contribute to bloating.

- **Probiotics:** Consider incorporating probiotics into your diet or as a supplement. Probiotics can help maintain a healthy balance of gut bacteria, potentially reducing gas and bloating.

- **Chew Food Slowly:** Eating slowly and mindfully can minimize the risk of swallowing excess air, which can lead to bloating and gas.

- **Stay Hydrated:** Drink plenty of water throughout the day to support digestion and prevent constipation, which can exacerbate bloating.

- **Regular Exercise:** Engaging in regular physical activity can help promote healthy digestion and reduce bloating. Even a short walk after a meal can be beneficial.

- **Over-the-Counter Remedies:** In some cases, over-the-counter gas-relief products may provide temporary relief from bloating and gas. Consult with a healthcare professional before using such products regularly.

It's important to work closely with a healthcare provider to develop a comprehensive plan for managing hiatal hernia symptoms. They can offer tailored advice and, if necessary, recommend medications or other interventions to alleviate your specific symptoms effectively.

CHAPTER 9

Lifestyle Changes for Hiatal Hernia

9.1 Weight Management

Maintaining a healthy weight is crucial for managing hiatal hernia symptoms. Excess weight, especially around the abdominal area, can increase pressure on the stomach and contribute to reflux. Here are some tips for weight management:

- **Healthy Diet:** Follow a balanced, hiatal hernia-friendly diet that focuses on portion control and nutrient-dense foods. Avoid overeating and limit high-fat or high-sugar foods.

- **Regular Exercise:** Engage in regular physical activity to help with weight management. Aim for a combination of cardiovascular exercise and strength training. Consult with a healthcare provider or a fitness professional to create a safe and effective exercise plan.

- **Hydration:** Stay well-hydrated with water and reflux-friendly beverages. Proper hydration can support overall health and help control appetite.

- **Monitor Caloric Intake:** Pay attention to your caloric intake and ensure that you're consuming an appropriate amount of calories for your activity level and weight goals.

- **Consult a Registered Dietitian:** Consider working with a registered dietitian who can provide personalized guidance on weight management and dietary choices specific to your needs.

9.2 Tips for Better Sleep

Getting quality sleep is essential for overall well-being and can significantly impact hiatal hernia symptoms. Here are some tips for improving your sleep:

- **Elevate Your Upper Body:** As mentioned earlier, elevate the head of your bed by 6-8 inches or use extra pillows to sleep at an incline. This position can help prevent nighttime reflux.

- **Finish Meals Early:** Finish your last meal at least 2-3 hours before bedtime to allow for proper digestion and reduce the risk of nighttime reflux.

- **Relaxation Techniques:** Practice relaxation techniques, such as deep breathing, meditation, or progressive muscle relaxation, before bedtime to reduce stress and promote better sleep.

- **Limit Fluid Intake:** While staying hydrated is important, reduce your fluid intake in the hours leading up to bedtime to minimize nighttime awakenings for bathroom trips.

- **Establish a Bedtime Routine:** Create a consistent bedtime routine to signal to your body that it's time to sleep. This routine can include activities like reading, taking a warm bath, or listening to soothing music.

- **Create a Comfortable Sleep Environment:** Ensure that your bedroom is conducive to sleep. Keep the room dark, quiet, and at a comfortable temperature. Invest in a supportive mattress and pillows.

- **Limit Caffeine and Alcohol:** Reduce or eliminate caffeine and alcohol intake, especially in the hours leading up to bedtime. Both can disrupt sleep patterns.

9.3 Stress Reduction

Stress can exacerbate hiatal hernia symptoms, so stress reduction techniques are essential for managing the condition. Here are some stress reduction strategies:

- **Mindfulness and Meditation:** Practice mindfulness and meditation to reduce stress and promote relaxation. These techniques can help you become more aware of your body and reduce muscle tension.

- **Yoga:** Incorporate yoga into your routine. Yoga combines physical postures, breathing exercises, and meditation to reduce stress and improve overall well-being.

- **Regular Exercise:** Engaging in
  regular physical activity can
  help reduce stress. Exercise
  releases endorphins, which are
  natural mood lifters.

- **Breathing Exercises:** Deep
  breathing exercises can be done
  anywhere and at any time to
  quickly reduce stress. Inhale
  deeply through your nose, hold
  the breath for a few seconds,
  and exhale slowly through your
  mouth.

- **Adequate Rest:** Ensure that
  you're getting enough quality
  sleep. Lack of sleep can
  contribute to stress, so
  prioritize good sleep hygiene.

- **Seek Support:** Consider
  speaking with a therapist or
  counselor to address any

emotional or psychological factors that may be contributing to stress.

- **Time Management:** Efficiently manage your time to reduce the pressure of rushed schedules and deadlines, which can contribute to stress.

- **Hobbies and Relaxation:** Engage in hobbies and activities that you enjoy to unwind and relax. This can be a great way to reduce stress and promote mental well-being.

Lifestyle changes are often a crucial component of managing hiatal hernia symptoms. Discuss these changes with a healthcare provider to ensure that they are tailored to your specific

needs and can effectively address
your symptoms and overall health.

www.ingramcontent.com/pod-product-compliance
Lightning Source LLC
Chambersburg PA
CBHW050833260726

48660CB00006B/2220